A DIET COOKBOOK FOR CROHN'S DISEASE

DESIGNING A DIET FOR PEOPLE WITH CROHN'S DISEASE

BRENDA DESKINS

Table of Contents

CHAPTER ONE

A DIET FOR CROHN'S DISEASE

Designing a Diet for People with Crohn's Disease

If you suffer from Crohn's disease, you may have noticed that certain foods bring on an intestinal flare. Your ability to self-manage your Crohn's disease, alleviate GI symptoms, and speed intestinal healing may depend on your familiarity with, and ability to avoid, these food triggers.

Similar to ulcerative colitis, it is a form of inflammatory bowel disease (IBD). These two conditions share the common thread of an immune response directed against the digestive system.

Crohn's disease is characterized by inflammation of the small intestine, which can result in gastrointestinal symptoms such as nausea, vomiting, diarrhea, and abdominal pain.

Inflammation reduces the body's ability to utilize the nutrients in the food you eat.

Absorptive difficulties may worsen after Crohn's surgery, in which a section of the intestine is removed.

Crohn's disease can make it difficult to eat well and stay at a healthy weight.

CHAPTER TWO

How Does One Create a Diet for Crohn's Disease?

You have likely read about the various Crohn's disease diets available. However, the reality is that there is no IBD diet that has been proven effective by science. However, many doctors believe that some patients, especially those experiencing acute attacks of their disease, can pinpoint specific foods that bring on their symptoms. Gas, bloating, abdominal pain, cramping, and diarrhea are all gastrointestinal (GI) symptoms that may be alleviated by avoiding your "trigger foods." You'll also be allowing your irritated digestive tract to rest and recover.

This is especially crucial during an acute episode of Crohn's disease symptoms. During a flare-up, it may be more taxing on your body to consume things like spicy or greasy foods, whole grains, high-fiber fruits and vegetables, nuts and seeds, caffeine, and alcohol.

Crohn's disease patients who have trouble absorbing nutrients should stick to a high-calorie, high-protein diet, even if it goes against their better judgment. Based on these considerations, an effective Crohn's disease diet plan would prioritize five or six meals per day, in addition to two or three snacks, as recommended by healthcare professionals. As a result, your intake of protein, calories, and other nutrients, in general, will be guaranteed. You should also take any vitamin and mineral supplements prescribed by your healthcare provider. You can restore lost nutrients in your body by doing this.

What should I not eat while on a diet for Crohn's disease?

Each person with Crohn's disease has a unique set of foods that bring on flare-ups. Identifying which foods, if any, cause yours will help you plan a healthy diet. Flare-ups of Crohn's disease are often made worse by eating any of the foods on the following list for many people. One or more of the following foods may be responsible for your symptoms:

• Alcohol (mixed drinks, beer, wine)

— Oils, butter, mayonnaise, and margarine

Beverages with Carbonation

• Caffeine, therba, and sweets

• Corn

The Dairy Industry (if lactose intolerant)

1. Fatty foods (fried foods)

high-fiber foods

Glutten-containing foods (lentils, beans, legumes, cabbage, broccoli, onions)

Seeds and nuts (peanut butter, other nut butters)

Foods that are eaten in their natural state, such as raw

Foods that are eaten in their raw state

* Beef and pork

Hot and spicy cuisine

Whole grains and bran

When you know which foods trigger your symptoms, you can either avoid them altogether or find ways to prepare them that reduce their impact. You'll have to try different foods and cooking techniques to find out what works for you. You may not have to completely cut out raw vegetables from your diet if they cause flare-ups. If you find that eating them raw causes gastrointestinal distress, try steaming, boiling, or stewing instead. You can try eating ground sirloin or ground round to see if you can tolerate a leaner cut of beef if you notice an increase in fat in the stools after consuming red meat. You could also choose to make fish or skinless, low-fat chicken your primary protein sources.

Can Crohn's Disease be Treated with a Diet Low in Residue?

Specific foods that contribute to stool residue are avoided on a low-residue diet. Stricture of the lower small intestine is a common symptom of Crohn's disease in people with small bowel involvement (the ileum). They may find relief from symptoms like diarrhea, cramping, and nausea by switching to a low-fiber, low-residue diet. Although there is a lack of conclusive evidence, it is possible that this diet could help some people have fewer bowel movements per week. On a low-residue diet, you might want to stay away from foods like:

• Corn cob husks

- Nuts

Foods that are eaten in their natural state, such as raw

- Seeds

Foods that are eaten in their raw state

CHAPTER THREE

Is There a Connection Between Crohn's Disease and Fiber?

The health benefits of a high-fiber diet cannot be overstated. Controlling your weight, blood pressure, and cholesterol levels can all benefit from this. In addition, consuming about 23 grams of fiber daily can reduce the likelihood of a Crohn's flare by as much as 40 percent. However, high-fiber foods may make your flare-up worse.

Soluble fiber foods are ideal for people with Crohn's disease. When there is too much fluid in the digestive tract, soluble fiber can help by soaking it up. Soluble fiber-rich foods have been shown to slow digestion and reduce diarrhea symptoms. Insoluble fiber, the other kind, can increase the amount of water present in the digestive tract. Foods will go through your system more quickly. Some of the possible side effects of that are watery diarrhea, abdominal cramping, and excessive gas. Too much insoluble fiber may lead to a blockage.

To get your daily dose of fiber, focus on plant-based fare. Fruits, vegetables, grains, beans, and nuts all fall under this category. Both soluble and insoluble fiber can be found in the majority of plant-based foods. To reduce insoluble fiber, wash produce thoroughly and remove peels, skin, and seeds. Look for added fiber on food labels, even in items like dairy.

Whenever you're not experiencing active Crohn's symptoms, go for whole grains and a wide variety of fresh fruits and vegetables.

Could keeping a food diary help me control my Crohn's disease?

Yes. If you keep a food diary, you may be able to pinpoint the "offenders" in your diet that are causing you problems. If your symptoms are particularly bad while your disease is active, avoiding these foods may help.

Keeping a food diary can help you and your doctor assess whether or not your diet is healthy and well-balanced. A sufficient amount of protein, carbohydrates, fats, and water can be measured. Whether or not you are getting enough calories to keep your weight and energy levels stable can also be determined.

Begin your food diary by keeping track of the foods you eat and the amounts you consume in a small notebook. Write the time, what you ate, and whether or not you experienced any adverse reactions in your notebook.

Consult with a dietitian after keeping a food diary for at least two weeks. The dietitian can tell you if you don't need to take any supplements because you're eating a healthy, balanced diet, or if you do. Healthy eating promotes self-healing and keeps you in good health. Your overall health and the management of Crohn's disease can benefit from a discussion about nutrition with a registered dietitian.

You may find that by avoiding certain foods that trigger disease symptoms, you are better able to manage their intensity and frequency when they occur. But don't impose such severe dietary restrictions on yourself that you exacerbate malnutrition, which frequently occurs in tandem with Crohn's disease. Find alternate means of obtaining the calories, protein, carbohydrates, and fats that you'll be missing from the foods you give up. That can be achieved by incorporating a diet rich in nutrients.

Although fast food is generally not recommended as part of a healthy diet, there are times when it can provide a much-needed nutritional boost. The calories and nutrients in some fast food options can be useful. Pizza, for instance, contains a variety of nutrients and calories, including protein, calcium, and vitamins A, B, C, and D. Calories and calcium both abound in a milkshake. Those who have lactose intolerance should take the necessary precautions before consuming any milk products.

Have a conversation with your doctor or nutritionist about taking vitamin and mineral supplements. Vitamin D deficiency is common, for instance, among those who suffer from Crohn's disease. Vitamin D in higher doses (1,000 to 2,000 IU daily) may be beneficial, according to a study published in the American Journal of Preventive Medicine. This may be especially true for lowering the risk of colorectal cancer, which may be elevated in those with IBD. The Vitamin D Reference Intake Level (2,000 IU/day) has been determined to be safe by the National Academy of Sciences. However, it is still recommended that you consult your physician to determine the correct dosage for you.

Am I able to manage my Crohn's disease symptoms with a liquid diet?

There is evidence that some people with Crohn's disease, particularly during a flare, may benefit from a high-calorie liquid diet, which supports the idea that liquid diets might help people with certain health conditions. Liquid diets can alleviate Crohn's disease symptoms by giving the digestive system a much-needed break. People with Crohn's disease who need extra nutrition on a temporary basis or who have intestinal malabsorption issues may benefit from the liquid diet or special high-calorie liquid formulas.

CHAPTER FOUR

In place of or in addition to your regular diet, you may drink liquid supplements like Ensure Plus or Boost Plus, which are part of the enteral nutrition system. A feeding tube can also be used to administer supplements in liquid form. When a child's growth has slowed or puberty has been delayed because of Crohn's disease, enteral nutrition is often helpful.

Bypassing your gut entirely with parenteral nutrition may be recommended in cases of severe flares, severe malnutrition, or small intestine loss due to surgery. An intravenous (IV) feed is a method of delivering fluid nutrients straight into the bloodstream via a catheter. This provides a rest for your intestines, which can reduce discomfort. The medical term for this is "bowel rest."

Do Omega-3 Fatty Acids and Probiotics Have Any Benefits?

Good fats, such as those found in fish oil and flaxseed oil, have been the subject of numerous studies that suggest they play a significant role in the inflammation associated with inflammatory bowel disease. However, it is unclear from the available research whether omega-3 fatty acids have any demonstrable anti-inflammatory effect on IBD. The addition of omega-3 fatty acid supplements to your diet should be discussed with your physician first.

Whether probiotics, or "good bacteria," can help with

gastrointestinal disorders like Crohn's disease and ulcerative colitis is the subject of a new line of research. However, more research is needed to confirm whether or not these supplements help promote intestinal healing in IBD.